# "Royal Melbourne Hospital and Associated Hospital School of Nursing"

*INTRODUCTION*

As a young nurse it was usual to commence training at the tender age of eighteen after completing the Victorian Year 12 (Matriculation) High School Certificate or its equivalent.

The "School of Nursing" was a revolutionary method of training as it incorporated on the job training whilst conducting "study blocks". These were held every three months at the college in Malvern Victoria, where nurses attended lectures 9-5pm, five days a week for a month. This procedure extended throughout the three years of training.

The lectures were given by doctors, pharmacists, physiotherapists and medical specialists representing their specific field of medicine. Assignments, assessments and examinations were held at the end of each "Block" session. Once back into one's base hospital we attended compulsory lectures weekly. In hospital we worked six days a week attending lectures, when scheduled, on or off duty.

During the three years training each nurse spent time at the "Royal Women's Hospital", 'The Royal Children's Hospital" and "Fairfield Infectious Diseases Hospital" with the majority of time spent at the home hospital, The Royal Melbourne Hospital.

For many years now there has been a debate regarding the "College training" versus "University training". Having observed, assessed and spoken to a large group of University trained nurses I cannot understand how the immersion method whereby experience was gained in the major specialist arena, could be improved upon. The practical work together with the theory seemed an ideal situation.

*An interesting aside:*
*During the period I am referring to there was also "The Teachers College" and "The Pharmacy College". It worked!*

Chapter 1

**It was different!**

Nursing is interesting, challenging and extremely satisfying.

*I have chosen to ponder about my time at Fairfield Hospital, for several reasons, mainly the unusual but interesting cases we experienced in a specific facility.*

My time spent training at Fairfield Hospital was memorable. It required all the skills we had as nurses to allay the fear of patients with unusual, often fatal diseases.

*Fairfield Infectious Diseases Hospital was originally known as Queens Memorial Infectious Diseases Hospital, operating from 1904 to 1996.*

The hospital was built on approximately fifteen acres of land on the banks of the Yarra River. The location was Fairfield which was a suburb of Melbourne, Victoria, Australia.

In the very late 1800's there was an overwhelming number of cases of infectious diseases. Diphtheria, Typhoid, Small Pox and Scarlet Fever were said to be problematic. At the time there were only a couple of major general hospitals and I understand a couple of specialist hospitals, a Children's and Eye and Ear Hospital.

This created an urgent need for another specialist hospital and so Victoria overcame the problem by converting an existing hospital into a specific Infectious diseases Hospital.

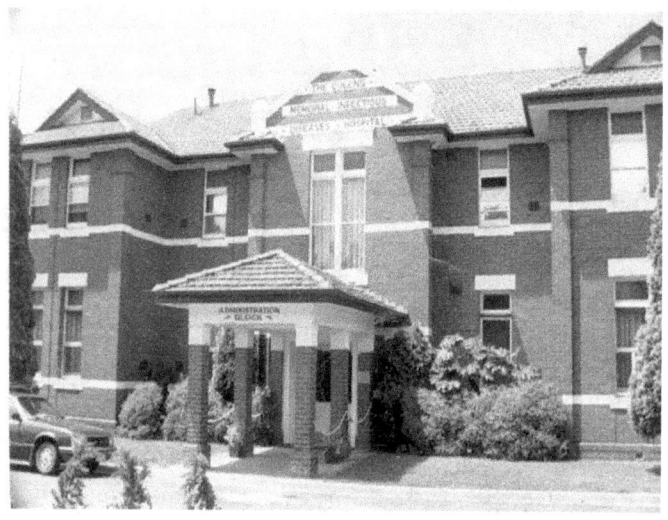

*Fairfield Infectious Diseases Hospital Administration Block*
*(Photo courtesy Darebin Libraries Victoria)*

Chapter 2

## Memories of Fairfield Hospital

My early memories of Fairfield Hospital are both happy and sad. Happy because as a young nurse I really loved the work I was doing. It was a completely "hands on" caring and interesting area of Public Health.

At the same time it was sad to see so many young people, during an outbreak of a disease, so sick and needing the skilled care and attention to get them through such a major event.

During the 1950's was a time when, in Australia, we had Tuberculosis, Diphtheria, Whooping Cough, and Poliomyelitis amongst other diseases, causing concern. Fairfield was at the "Cutting edge" of education, research and treatment of infectious diseases.

The land surrounding Fairfield Hospital was at the time, a large amount of land with trees and shrubs and was basically isolated. The entrance off the road was gated and permanently manned twenty four hours a day. A uniformed man would exit his wooden building-office to enquire about the business of the visitors. Were they visiting patients were they indeed patients themselves or staff. Depending on reply the visitor would be directed to their intended destination.

Further along the road was a separate entrance, not formally identified, however the adjoining land was deliberately tucked back making it difficult to view as there was a dwelling that housed patients with Leprosy, later known as Hansen's disease.

Rumours ran rife back then in the 1950's. "Leprosy" was regarded as an exotic disease. Research was being conducted and little said until more was known.

Fear of an emotive reaction from the public was uppermost in the authorities' minds. To prevent public outcry "Leprosy" was not written or talked about during this period! Only medical staff really knew what exactly was in-house at any time. Not all general staff needed in-depth details about the varied infectious diseases housed in the institution. This was not secrecy, as such, however we were dealing with an emotive issue at the time and The Public Health System was not necessarily understood by the lay-man.

In general the patients who came to Fairfield Hospital had either been too difficult to diagnose, required specialist treatment or were a risk to the general public and therefore required admission to a central facility. The world was becoming a smaller world as travellers could get from country to country in less time, allowing infectious diseases to incubate during travel. *After* getting to our shores they often presented with a "full blown" disease, not usually present in Australia.

Fairfield Infectious Diseases Hospital, as a stand-alone hospital received patients from all states of Australia and included South East Asia when and if specialist treatment was required.

Australia had Quarantine Stations dotted around the country in areas where airports and seaports were the points of entry for visitors from overseas. These stations were in areas of isolation, patients were assessed and those that required hospitalisation were sent on to Fairfield Hospital.

Quarantine, at that time, was effective, it was efficient and a necessary border protection for Australia.

CHAPTER 3

*Admission:*

Most patients arrived by ambulance, others by car after pre-arranged admission with their doctors. On arrival patients were usually admitted to the "F.G. Scholes Block" built around 1947. This was a three story brick building. Each floor having single rooms and each room had a small gauzed veranda. The rooms were light, bright, sufficiently roomy and very well designed for practicality, efficiency and maximum prevention of contamination or cross-infection.

Each room had a radio and airy surrounds, no air-conditioning of course. However this was Melbourne, Victoria and the grounds backed on to the Yarra River. Green lawns and shady trees surrounding the buildings thus a very pleasant temperature ensured.

On admission the patient was allocated a bedroom on the Ground to 3rd Floor. The patient, child or adult was bed-bathed, hair was washed and fine tooth-combed, body examined for sores, bruises or cuts.

Observations were taken and all information was recorded in a patient's personal file. Basic assessment completed, numerous pathology tests were undertaken, X-Rays if applicable were carried out.

ALL procedures were performed in the isolation of the block. While the patient's diagnosis was being confirmed, visitors were restricted and the patient was *treated as infectious.* They therefore remained in isolation.

Outside each patient's room a clear plastic holder was attached to the wall beside the door into the room. For all using the hallway the card holder was obvious. Room number, Name of patient and a Coloured Card were on display. A blue card or a blue card with red stars indicated the degree-severity of infectiousness. The degree of caution required by those who entered the room was signified by the number of Stars displayed on the Blue Card System.

*Plain blue card* represented mildly infectious therefore basic cleanliness-hygiene was required to prevent cross-infection.

**Examples:**     Hansen's disease, Tetanus, Tuberculosis, Gas-Gangrene

*On entry to room the procedure was to wash hands at basin with antiseptic solution. Hibitane and Zephirin were both being used at the time.*

*Blue card* **with one red star** usually indicated a lot more caution required.

**Example:**     Measles, Mumps, Chicken Pox, Croup, Whooping Cough

*When entering a room hand washing at basin with the addition of a gown and removal before leaving room.*

*Blue card with two red stars* indicated a seriously infectious disease where all prevention must be taken.

**Example:**     Diphtheria, Poliomyelitis, Tape Worm, Hook Worm Exotic-Island worm infestations-diseases

*When entering a room the procedure beginning with hand washing at basin with the addition of a gown and gloves all removed before leaving room.*

**The highest of all, a blue card with three red stars** indicated the highest degree of infectiousness.

**Example:**     Smallpox, Typhoid

*When entering a room hand washing at basin with the addition of a gown and gloves. Also all hair undercover and mask to be worn at all times.*

*All **medical staff required** protective clothing over street uniform-dress covering. This was precautionary and needed to be carefully removed before leaving the room. Room and contents to be treated with extreme caution, keeping in mind the ease of picking up and carrying on infection.*

Patients' food was brought up from the kitchens situated elsewhere on the grounds. The meals were on trays, labelled with name and ward number. The nursing staff took **from** the trolley **to** the patient and **from** the patient **to** the trolley. Not a job left to the catering or kitchen staff. All food left over was dumped into large, tight lidded receptacles placed in the kitchenette, next to the entrance to the ward.

ALL left over food was to be destroyed to prevent cross-infection.

ALL **clean** linen was taken to the laundry department on the grounds, in huge canvas bags with tie-tops.

ALL **dirty-soiled** linen was placed in stainless steel bins with tight fitting lids that contained *PHENYLE*. Linen was soaked for a pre-determined period of time using a certain strength of diluted Phenyl before being taken out of the ward to the laundry.

Pans were also stainless steel. Once collected they were delivered to the pan-room, emptied, flushed then placed into the huge sterilizers constantly kept on the boil. Any pans from **3 Star rooms** were placed, with contents, into lidded containers and soaked in *PHENYLE* before being emptied, flushed then placed in sterilisers.

*Imagine.... cross-infection was negligible to non-existent, an amazing record and proof that the Barrier Nursing routine-ritual worked!!!*

CHAPTER 4

*Minimising Cross-Infection:*

Throughout the grounds were mostly single but up to three story stand-alone buildings and each would take approximately thirty patients. They were positioned with considerable space surrounding each. Overhanging shady trees and lawns surrounded the buildings and large open verandas were wrapped around the four sides.

The theory was, to minimize cross-infection it was essential to give the patient abundant fresh air and sunshine and to create an imaginary barrier; and a haven of peacefulness.

After a patient's disease was confirmed (usually in the block) they were then transferred to a relevant area within the hospital. If one was confirmed with tuberculosis, after the initial period of illness, the patient was transferred to the TB Ward where management focused on medication, strict rest, physiotherapy and a nutritious diet.

Croup, Whooping Cough and Diphtheria were admitted, if referred to Fairfield after confirmation of diagnosis, to a single dwelling building which housed thirty patients. Often these patients by-passed "The Block" and were admitted directly to the specific ward.

The design was such that the two Tracheostomy Theatres were in the centre of the building adjacent to the Nurses Station to enable close monitoring.

Each theatre was set up as an operating theatre but could also be converted to a "Steam Room". A large ground-planted container, with a "Flue" attached, belched out a vapour of steam and "Fryers Balsam". The moist air circulating into the single room assisted the patient to breathe more easily.

If any sign of an emergency such as respiration compromised, the patient was already in an emergency theatre where an incision was made on the patient's throat, over the trachea, an airway was inserted to enable the person to breathe again. With lungs expanding, oxygen was again circulated to the major organs of the body.

*CHAPTER 5*

*<u>Note</u>: This chapter will cover a few of the most common diseases admitted to Fairfield Hospital during the only period I feel equipped to speak about.*

*The period between 1950's and early 1960's I had first-hand knowledge and on the spot observation, however the remarks are purely from my personal experiences.*

## POLIOMYELITIS OUTBREAK

**Poliomyelitis** (Infantile Paralysis) A Viral infection.

Poliomyelitis attacked a large number of children. Many of whom were infants. Those in their early teens seemed to be the majority. I also saw a reasonable number of early twenty year olds, yet older people were less inclined to be attacked and the elderly rarely succumbed to the disease.

There were several Poliomyelitis **outbreaks** during my time at Fairfield Hospital, and as explained previously the patients were admitted to the Block where the routine Admissions Procedure was carried out, a room allocated and the patient's treatment progressed from there.

When a Poliomyelitis patient's condition was deemed no longer infectious the patient went one of two ways.

One way was to be transferred to a ground floor ward where the focus was on intensive Physiotherapy, Occupational Therapy, a healthy diet, rest and fresh air (anything to assist with a patient's recovery).

*Compromised breathing*: The patient whose breathing was affected and respiratory muscles compromised was placed in a separate building where there were fifteen respirators down each end of the ward. The male and female wards were separated by a Nurses Station.

Each respirator was attached to a hose that went through the wall and the other end joined together with the bellows. The mechanical movement of the machines was strictly maintained. Each motor-bellows was connected to an emergency backup power system. It all worked well.

The respirators were reasonably noisy, a hum that became very familiar. It was a sound associated with security and safety, always there in the background…. comforting.

Junior nurses, new to Fairfield, often reported the sound to be quite eerie at night when walking to the Nurses' Home along the pathways with shadows from tree branches, scuffling of possums and the hum of the motors! It was suggested by the "old guard" to stare straight ahead, hold your breath and manage a quick walk, as running was a definite **No-No**!

The respirators otherwise known as Iron-Lungs were the size of a *narrow* single bed with a mattress. A lid enclosed the entire contraption. At the top end was an opening where the patient's head was protruding and a soft collar (rubber gasket) surrounded the neck to allow an internal vacuum!

The mechanical action of the bellows was to pump air in and out of the Iron-Lung. When the air went in it would create a gentle pressure around the chest and the patient would exhale. Then when the air was pumped out it would drop the pressure enabling the patient to breathe in through their nose and mouth.

A wonderful invention, a gentle but sustainable solution to respiratory paralysis. Simply the difference in air-pressure resulting in a mechanical action......enabling a satisfactory breathing style.

To be in a respirator was in itself a sign of the precariousness of the medical condition. Each patient required intensive nursing. The Iron-Lungs were cumbersome for actual nursing. Access to the patient was awkward and slow, particularly when personal hygiene was needed frequently with access to the bottom sheet required. This included attention to bowels and bladder and straightening underneath sheet to prevent creases causing a "rub area on the skin". Bed baths and massaging pressure-points regularly helped minimize skin-breaks, thus keeping the immobile patient as healthy as possible.

Access to the respirators was also frequently required by the Physiotherapists. They needed to attend to the muscles to minimize the flaccid state of the extremities attention was also required in an attempt to re-educate the limbs.

The patients each had fixed to the frame, a medium size mirror, this was clamped to the top lid of the respirator. This fixture enabled wider vision for the patient. They could see around the ward, minimising the feeling of isolation. Their situation was mostly long term and it was vitally important for the patient to have visual access to as much around them as possible. In fact, vital to be part of their environment.

For longer term patients, we were able to position a book for them to read, like a chant one would hear in the background *"Page nurse"* and whoever was walking past would detour to *turn the page* for the patient.


***Non-compromised breathing***: The patient whose breathing wasn't compromised was in a bed in a Polio-General Ward. This ward was a-buzz with activity. The physiotherapists worked one on one routinely and regularly to minimise the constriction of the muscles, a painful process for the patient.

The endless massaging and exercising both passive and active was an important part of re-educating the muscles. This procedure strengthened the muscles and sent signals through to the brain teaching the body to effectively regain and utilise movement. Re-educating a patient's body, to re-establish some movement was a slow, tedious process. The movement they had previously often seemed elusive, causing a diverse range of emotions.

The emotional health of the patient was critical to the speed of recovery.

Some patients had Stryker Frames, a wonderful device which provided the patient with a frame to prevent distortion. A patient would be placed into the frame in-between sessions and removed from the frame when activity was required and procedures were underway.

The Bradford frame was also in use, however there had been a great deal of discussion regarding the Kenny versus Conventional method of treatment. To the best of my recollection during my time we used a combination of both methods.

There was a leaning towards gentle movement together with moist warm compresses as opposed to total immobilization....and it worked, our recovery rate was impressive.

During rest times in the afternoon and when preparing patients for overnight, the patients were placed back into their frames and bandaged into position to prevent any limb movement not considered to be a natural position.

The movements of patients' limbs often caused distress, thus it was important for the mood of the overall ward to be positive and caring. Working with the physiotherapists, were occupational therapists and dieticians as it was imperative to build up the health of the mind and body. A complete approach was essential, now days referred to as a holistic approach.

Nurses worked closely with each of these ancillary specialists. The nurses were the primary carers and were required to carry on the specialists' work around the clock, seven days a week. It was intensive treatment with mainly wonderful results.

Our patients were long term and as nurses we were instructed to remain professional at all times; the patient was a priority. We were continuously reminded that our personal feelings were not to encroach or intrude on the firm, confident and positive manner that was normally demonstrated when interacting with patients.

It was often difficult to emotionally ignore the insecurities voiced by many of the older patients. There were fathers and mothers each unsure of their futures and children scared of being away from home. The psychological trauma was indescribable for many, therefore so important for us, the nurses, to continue caring, but remain strong and confident.

*The training we the nurses received managed to squeeze from our willing bodies the attributes so necessary to continue day after day. Interestingly we are talking about young ladies as young as eighteen years of age!*

With the discipline that was "dished out" and the behaviour that was expected, the response to such an authoritive environment was truly a result of the times in which we lived…..The -1950's.

*In hindsight nursing was a vocation…..certainly not a job.*
*Once a nurse always a nurse!*

*Note:*
*The discovery of Salk vaccine and Sabin vaccine in the 1950's eventually saw Poliomyelitis eradicated from Australia.*

CHAPTER 6

*MAJOR INFECTIOUS DISEASES PRESENTING 1950-1965*
*TUBERCULOSIS*

**Tuberculosis** –This disease is caused by the Tubercle Bacillus.

A brief description (to help understanding, as this is not a technical book). In human Tuberculosis there is Pulmonary Tuberculosis and Extra-Pulmonary Tuberculosis.

Pulmonary Tuberculosis = Chronic Adult Type and Acute Pulmonary Tuberculosis

Extra-Pulmonary Tuberculosis - Occurs in many different forms some not as common as others:

- TB of the Bones and Joints
- TB of the Glands
- TB Peritonitis, Meningitis, Renal
- TB Laryngitis

The diagnosis of Tuberculosis is multi-faceted. The most important part is to isolate the bacillus of course...difficult.

Tuberculosis is common in so many countries. Many people have been exposed to the bacilli therefore a positive Mantoux test is not a stand-alone diagnosis at all. The test simply indicates having been exposed to the disease.

Fluid from Pleural cavities, Gastric Lavage, Cerebrospinal fluid, Urine and X-rays to name a few, are the important tests carried out on a patient's admission to hospital.

It must be emphasised that Tuberculosis is a serious disease and one not to under estimate, remembering that this disease wasn't as common in Australia as many of the overseas countries at that time.

After time spent in the "Block" undergoing tests the patient was then sent to the Rehabilitation-Tuberculosis wards, on site, prior to an eventual transfer to a Sanatorium.

Patients arrived from the "block" when their condition was confirmed to be at a stage of extremely low infectiousness. They continued with their prescribed treatment, once again requiring regular physiotherapy. The sight of patients hanging over the sides of their beds with nurses and physios pummelling their backs to loosen the mucous in their chests was a sight to see!

The most common Tuberculosis I remember nursing was the Pulmonary Tuberculosis.

Many of these patients came from an area recognised as, an immigration re-settlement facility and many had arrived in

Victoria direct from various overseas migrant camps. It was reported at the time that their previous close-living and less than healthy conditions, lack of food and more importantly poor nutrition was a breeding ground for Tuberculosis.

The incubation period of Tuberculosis was said to be 21-28 days. By the time people were evacuated from the overseas facility, mainly by ship which was a slow trip, they would be likely to be incubating the disease ready to start showing signs and symptoms of the infection after arrival in Australia.

The continuous low grade fever, night sweats, fatigue, breathlessness, lack of appetite and constant cough resulted in thin, gaunt and unwell patients. The depth of coughing would rack their already weak bodies but the blood spotted sputum would generally un-nerve the bravest amongst them.

The junior nurses on morning shift would collect the labelled stainless steel sputum mugs routinely changed, take them out to the pan-room and count the pieces (of sputum) plugs of mucous coughed up overnight, then record the results. We would graph the results each day enabling us to see improvement or otherwise.

Medication, rest, nutritious food, fresh-air and sunshine were of primary importance. Reduction of night sweats and a feeling of wellness combined to enable the patient's preparedness for transfer to a Sanatorium - Nursing Home That was dependant on the medical observations, which required a consistently normal temperature, maintained for a suitable period, and pathological results which were acceptable and supported the patients overall condition.

The mobile patients enjoyed the treed grounds and the attractively set out gardens which progressed their recovery....preparing them for the next step in their preparation for recovery.

Note: During the late 1940's an immunization program was introduced. BCG or Bacilli Calmette-Guerin was used nationally and given if a negative result to the Mantoux test. This was given as a part of a preventative program, remaining in effect until about the 1980's and ceased following the steep decline of Tuberculosis.

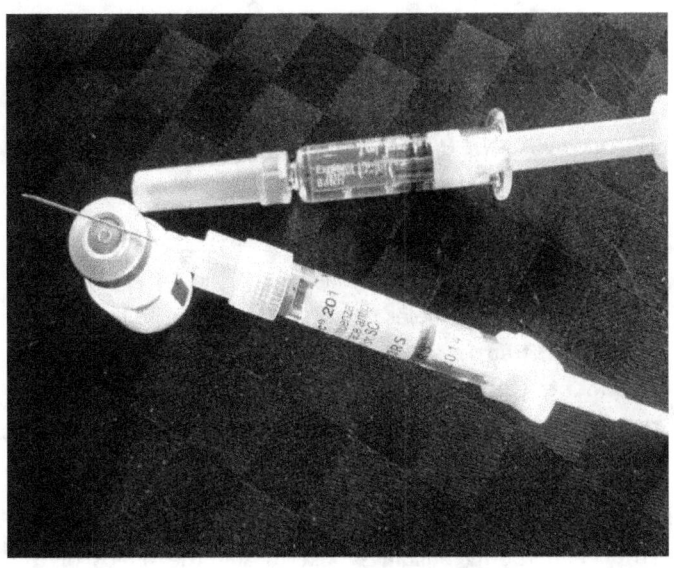

*Immunisation was compulsory and effective during my time at Fairfield Hospital.*

*CHAPTER 7*

*MAJOR INFECTIOUS DISEASES PRESENTING 1950-1965*

**WHOOPING-COUGH, SCARLET FEVER, CROUP and DIPTHERIA:**

For all admissions of the above diseases the procedure previously referred to was followed. Again, after the initial admission to the "Scholes Block", once diagnosed the patient would be transferred to the outer wards for ongoing treatment. This method of isolation, tests, diagnosis then distribution-transfer to the specific ward was an incredibly smart way of preventing cross-infection.

The outer wards were of similar design, airy, mainly one story, and roomy buildings built to suit the needs of the specific patients directed to this particular area. However the inside design was a little different. In the centre of the multi-purpose ward was the Nurses-Station arranged to view all within.

For a patient with *Croup, Whooping Cough, Scarlet Fever or Diphtheria*, the set up was ideal. On each side of the station was a mini-theatre set up for an emergency operation. Each theatre was a mirror image of the other. The lights, theatre bed, instrument trolley, cylinders of oxygen and nitrous oxide were tucked near the wall with masks and tubing within easy reach.

A glass partition separated the theatre bed from a large cot beside which was a HUGE kettle like container. It was used to hold hot water. We would pour "Friar's Balsam" on the top of the simmering water, encouraging the steam to fill this section, helping to loosen phlegm and relieve the breathing of the patients in distress. The steam expectantly would loosen the obstructing membrane from across the trachea and in many instances prevent the need for a tracheostomy.

A Tracheostomy is an emergency surgical procedure, used to insert an airway into a patient's throat to save a life. This metal tube allows the nurse to "suck out" the membrane or phlegm enabling an unhindered airway and it also allowed oxygen to be given to the patient directly into the lungs.

*Scarlet Fever* –Haemolytic Streptococcus

Often causing restrictive to insufficient air into the lungs and could require intervention. Once again high temperature, rash and a reasonably ill patient. However the area we mostly observed was the function of the kidneys, therefore regular collection, testing and reporting of urinary specimens was vital.

*Whooping-Cough* – Pertussis – Pertussis Bacillus

Caused by an organism called pertussis bacillus. It was agonising for all within hearing distance to be near these distraught children. The ages affected seemed to be very young children including little babies. It was so distressing.

We had oxygen bottles beside each cot-bed and on the locker an oxygen mask and nasal prongs.

The sound was hard on the staff. We tried to be clinical but to see little ones going from a blue tinge to navy blue was a stressful time. Each of us staff members would, for comfort, carry a baby over our shoulder whilst attending to others. I believed that an upright position, gently patting their back and being held firmly helped comfort them a little. The "Whoop" was the sound made after coughing whereby the patient was endeavouring to get a gulp of air.

Once the antibiotics, moist air, calm attitude combined it enabled the cough to settle thus lessening anxiety.

### Croup (Laryngo-Tracheo-Bronchitis or LTB)

It was thought that it was a viral infection. Treatment being much the same as for Diphtheria, requiring moist warm air and occasionally a tracheostomy to assist breathing if the pharyngeal area becomes too swollen. Laryngitis usually occurred with a sore throat and other wretched upper respiratory symptoms. Breathing difficulties were relieved by the warm moist air.

Croup is spread by the spray of droplets in the air from coughing or nasal discharge and mucous, hence all routine Barrier Nursing was required. Treated similarly to the other respiratory illnesses from a nursing point of view. Distressing.

### Diphtheria – Diphtheria bacillus (K.L.B)

Diphtheria had become uncommon in the late 50's early 1960's as immunisation was available and thankfully accessed, preventing major outbreaks.

However we occasionally had a case admitted. The patient was always very ill to need to be hospitalised. Incubation is short, around two to three days. It is only moderately infectious and nowhere near as infectious as measles or chicken-pox for example. The most common method of spread is by carrier, infection especially from nasal discharge. When looking for a carrier nasal and throat swabs are taken for evidence of infection.

The severity of the case is determined by the amount of toxins produced, the position of the membrane, whether it is nasal, tonsillar, nasopharyngeal or elsewhere, dictates the effect on breathing therefore the need of a tracheotomy.

The patient could be hospitalised for months. They are usually very sick especially if the amount of toxaemia is great and particularly so with nasopharyngeal cases.

The toxicity affects the body, more particularly the cardiovascular system. This is about as serious as it gets. Skilled nursing is required as Sulphonamides are said to have no effect on the disease. Antibiotics are mainly useful for carriers. The staff were periodically swabbed and if we were found to have a positive nasal swab we were given

Streptomycin cream to be inserted into the nostrils until a negative result was returned!

**All sources state there is <u>no excuse</u> for home-grown Diphtheria as immunisation is available to all.**

*CHAPTER 8*

*MAJOR INFECTIOUS DISEASES PRESENTING 1950-1965*

**MEASLES, MUMPS, CHICKEN POX:**

*Patients were admitted using the same admissions procedure, initially into "The Block" because in most instances if a patient needed hospitalisation with Measles or Chicken Pox it would usually be because of complications or needing isolation due to living arrangements.*

**Measles** (A Virus) a nasty disease, making the patient feel wretched, with temperature, aches and flue like symptoms. A rash, if inside the mouth and the entire gut it certainly will make one feel miserable. Mostly a phobia to light is present as measles can cause sore red eyes, the rash can affect the lungs and airways but mainly causes pneumonia as a secondary complication. Once the immune system catches up and the antibiotics kick in, the patient can usually go home with instructions that will keep them on the road to recovery by paying attention to nutrition, rest and fresh air.

*Mumps* (Parotitis) was another infectious and painful contractible disease. During the incubation period the patient would often display febrile condition, runny nose, sore throat and swelling of the parotid gland (the right and or the left side of the area in front of the ear lobe) and areas around the mandible (jaw). The swelling would continue down the side of the neck usually affecting swallowing and neck movement.

Mumps was a complaint that concerned the male adult and teenager as a reasonably serious complication, Orchitis, was known to affect the testicles. Heralded by a spike in temperature and a reddened, swollen genital area, it is said to be quite painful. It must be regarded as a serious complication that can cause sterilisation-infertility.

*Chicken-Pox* (Varicella) can progress from high temperature, runny nose, and nasty blisters to debilitating complications. On arrival the patient may have pustules that are weeping and itchy, in the eyes and mouth as well as affecting the mucous membrane. This of course would affect the gastrointestinal tract.

The sores-pustules can become infected, from scratching primarily. Luke warm baths, not too hot, containing sodium bicarbonate followed with a pat-dry as opposed to a rub dry, would sometimes ease the itch! We also used Calamine Lotion to dab on sores for the cooling and anti-itching effect.

However the greatest fear was always Encephalitis, an inflammation of the surrounding areas of the brain. With this potential complication, a Chicken-Pox patient would have a temperature, headache and become progressively drowsy over a period of time and begin to show signs of being difficult to rouse. If this serious complication arose it was usually a week after the "main event", an unexpected and unfortunate turn-around when one was expecting improvement.

On admission, if a diagnosis-medical history made one suspect Encephalitis a lumbar puncture would be performed. This medical procedure was performed in the patient's room under **sterile conditions**. The doctor administered a local anaesthetic to the lumbar region and then inserted a wide bored needle and gently tapped into the spinal fluid.

The Cerebrospinal Fluid collected could then be grown in a suitable medium by the Pathologist to confirm the diagnosis.

After confirmation the patient would be treated with antibiotics either orally or intravenously, which ever was appropriate at the time.

The patient was regarded as infectious until the last pustule dried and fell off.

Pneumonia can also be a secondary complication of Chicken-Pox. This too would require antibiotics and general nursing to build up basic health.

*CHAPTER 9*

*MAJOR INFECTIOUS DISEASES PRESENTING 1950-1965*

### INFECTIOUS HEPATITIS, ANTHRAX, TETANUS:

*Infective Hepatitis* (A Virus), patients diagnosed with Hepatitis were frequently admitted mainly by ambulance, or arriving pre-arranged with a referral from attending private doctor. These patients were admitted to the "Scholes Block" where the routine admissions procedure was undertaken.

Pathology would require blood, faeces and urine specimens to be collected for confirmation of disease and to establish the degree of seriousness.

The Dietician would immediately be notified as diet played an incredibly important part of treatment and recovery. Patients were served "Low Fat" diets and food was carefully monitored.

The patient's skin was usually itchy from the bilirubin (crystals settling on the skin) and the conjunctiva of the eyes were yellow. Jaundice continued to spread over the body.

The liver if compromised and being such an important organ needed to be accurately tracked to record stages of improvement. These patients were usually quite ill and *highly infectious*. The patients required isolation and careful monitoring to prevent further damage to the liver. Recovery was slow, these patients required close attention.

**Anthrax** (Bacillus anthracic) this was a disease rarely seen by me but occasionally we admitted patients with Anthrax. We knew it as Wool-sorters' disease as it was actually a disease of cattle and sheep, however men working in the industry could acquire Anthrax by inhaling the spores that were in the dust of the skins and wool.

The spores could live for years. The prognosis was never very positive as the respiratory system was usually severely affected. Anthrax had a high mortality rate in the 1950's.

**Tetanus** (Tetanus Bacillus) this disease affects the central nervous system causing very painful spasms of the muscles. During my time I witnessed several severe cases of tetanus.

We were aware that Tetanus was caused by a powerful nerve toxin produced by the an-aerobic bacillus that lives in manured farming land. I have seen a few cases and all came from agricultural areas. It was, at that time, said to live in a horse's gut.

In a particularly serious-advanced case I "Specialled" that is dedicated my time to the one person for not only continuity but special care. I was with this child who went into spasm with the slightest movement or noise. We had external signs *demanding* "QUIET" down passage ways, walk ways and within areas surrounding his room. He was a special case indeed.

We kept this lad who was such a severe case, sedated using muscle relaxants. With severe convulsions an Anaesthetist would induce sleep. A tracheostomy was required and the patient was ventilated.

Tetanus was a disease we admitted rarely. Interestingly it is a disease that the majority of the population understands, without argument, the benefits from immunisation.

A very toxic nerve toxin is produced by the bacilli which attacks the central nervous system. This in turn affects the muscles, particularly the jaw and mouth giving the disease the name "Lockjaw".

The specific treatment, at the time was Tetanus antitoxin together with sedation and muscle relaxants. The patients were kept sedated sometimes for weeks.

Expert supervision was needed as the muscle relaxants would affect the respiration, thus requiring not only tracheostomy but ventilation.

Now days most people are **up to date with Tetanus immunization** and in cases of a visit to Casualty are often given a booster injection.

*Interestingly, I have* <u>*not*</u> *met many people who have actually nursed a patient with Tetanus.* ***A frightening disease, now rarely seen due to immunisation.***

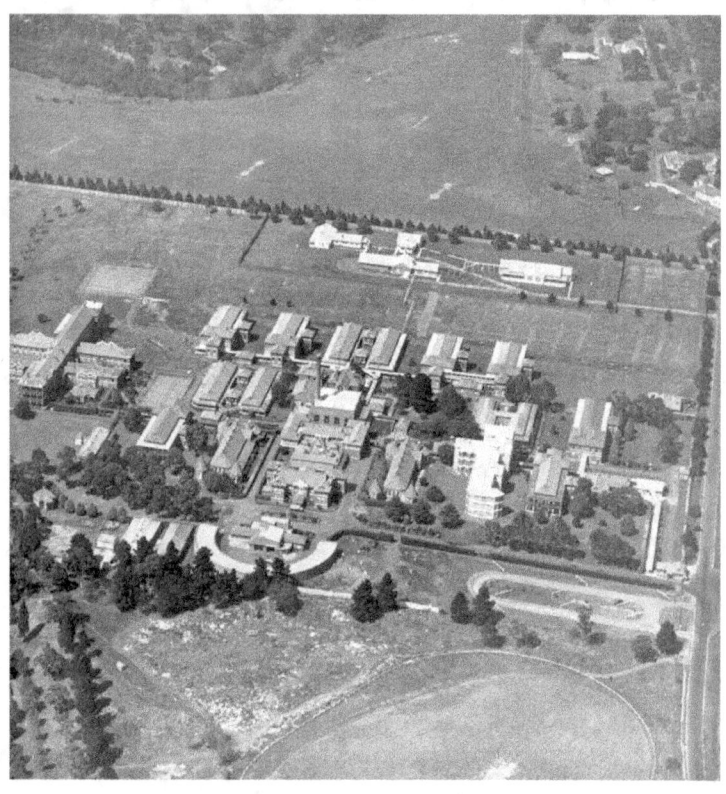

Aerial Photo of Fairfield Infectious Diseases Hospital
(Photo courtesy Darebin Libraries Victoria)

CHAPTER 10

*EXOTIC DISEASES:*

Gas-Gangrene......A disease that was extremely rare and mostly fatal.

***Gas-Gangrene*** (Clostridia) I only remember a couple of cases.

A patient was transferred from "The Snowy Mountain Scheme" where he had been working using massive tunnel digging machinery. It seems that somehow he or his clothing became caught in the mechanics of a powerful belt that moved the overburden. Staff finally extracted him from this terrible accident.

It appeared that his shoulder and arm were being dragged causing his body to be implicated further so that his head was also exposed to the heat and friction of the belt. The friction burnt through exposing his skull

We were advised later that we were to receive a transfer from another hospital to prepare for a seriously ill man. This man was being transferred to Fairfield with critical injuries. Ultimately this man had developed Gas Gangrene, an infection that affects the deep muscles, usually resulting from severe trauma. The bacteria releases toxins and produces gas which is trapped deep in the tissues.

I nursed this very ill man. The smell associated with this disease is peculiar to Gas Gangrene and once experienced it is a smell that one could identify anywhere at any time. (Another reason to actually nurse these unusual cases; the physical experience cannot be gotten from theory alone)

**Small-Pox** (A Virus) it was referred to as the most infectious of all diseases. It has caused widespread epidemics in certain tropical countries. Massive numbers died as a result of the epidemics.

During the 1950's Small Pox was not overly common in Australia however patients were admitted mainly from trading ships and other travellers arriving at our shores.

*Very few severe outbreaks have been experienced in countries where vaccinations are **accessed.***

I remember cases admitted to Fairfield Hospital because of the virulence associated with this disease. The recovery was slower also, as patients were isolated until the pustules-scabs had separated and scars healed.

The nursing of these patients required absolute skill. There was no cure at the time. The condition included such a severe febrile condition that hallucinations were frequently experienced and complications were common.

*Typhoid Fever* (Bacillus Typhosis) is spread through lack of sanitation, contamination of water or food and is more common in areas where there is overcrowding as in camps for people fleeing war-zones.

Once again we had a few cases however they were brought in to Australia through travel or immigration. The patients required strict isolation. All bedpans were soaked in 1-10 Lysol for several hours prior to further sterilisation.

The patients I remember with Typhoid were young men transferred from cargo ships who had been very healthy prior to being struck down with Typhoid. It was certainly an extremely debilitating disease with high temperatures for several days and diarrhoea. I remember a drug called Chloramphenicol being all that was available some sixty years ago.

Intestinal tract perforation, haemorrhage and heart failure are very real outcomes if careful nursing and suitable medication are not administered.

Rehabilitation was slow and the patient was not released from isolation alone until the faeces and urine were free from the typhoid bacilli.

*Meningitis* (Meningococcal, pneumococcal-influenzal, streptococcal, staphylococcal and various pus forming organisms) There is also, Viral and Tuberculus Meningitis.

This is a disease causing an inflammation of the meninges which causes intracranial pressure. The signs and symptoms are typical of this pressure. The patients we admitted were quite seriously ill and were showing symptoms of neck rigidity, headache, mild temperature, vomiting progressing through to convulsions. A haemorrhagic rash may also occur.

A lumbar puncture was urgently undertaken on admission as isolating and identifying the organism in the cerebrospinal fluid was the important step in successfully treating the patient.

All told, very ill patients of all ages were admitted to Fairfield Hospital regularly as a complication to an infectious disease or because of a pus forming organism of several types.

Meningococcus Bacteria was the most common cause of Meningitis during the 1950-60's. A very serious disease.

On the other hand it appeared that viral meningitis, was seen in clusters and associated with seasons of the year. Therefore it was my observation that more patients were seen in Autumn-Winter during my time at Fairfield Hospital.

CHAPTER 11

## TROPICAL OR SUB-TROPICAL DISEASES

**Malaria** is caused by a parasite called the plasmodium. The malarial parasite is passed on to humans by an infected mosquito (Anopheles Mosquito).

During my time at Fairfield we regularly admitted patients who had either visited countries where Malaria occurred or they were patients who were here to be treated. Sometimes the patient was not diagnosed when we admitted them but were showing all the signs and symptoms of an "infectious disease".

The patient's high temperatures, profuse sweating, severe rigors and headaches to name a few of the symptoms were evident but it was not until the specimen of blood confirmed the presence of the parasite that treatment could commence

Education programs were regularly rolled-out, for without utilising the medication available to prevent malaria it was not only a re-occurring and debilitating disease but also prevalent in the tropical areas.


**Leprosy** otherwise known as Hansen's disease was caused by a Bacillus. During my time it was feared by the general public.

Fairfield Hospital housed a certain number of patients on the 15 acres of land. Separated from the main buildings and as far away as possible was an area that housed these patients in buildings unseen from the road, or in fact the main hospital.

Rumours floated around but very few of us actually nursed there. A couple of nurses in our group did a stint in the "unmentionable" section but little was said! The paranoia was such that even our colleagues were advised not to discuss the ward. It was impressed on us that leprosy had an incubation period of 2-20 years. It was spread by sputum, nasal discharge or skin surrounding the ulcerated areas.

Today it is known as reasonably easy to treat, mainly confined to certain countries and not common enough to be of great concern.

I find it amazing comparing the difference in the acceptance by the general public now to sixty plus years ago.

*Cholera* (Vibrio Comma Bacillus) is an extremely serious disease and often fatal. I only remember a few cases admitted to Fairfield, once again patients visiting our shores.

I guess the reason we didn't see many cases in Australia is the origin of an outbreak is usually amongst homeless, prisoner of war camps, refugee camps and areas where people are living in squalid conditions.

Australia didn't have the conditions required for Cholera to thrive. It is so infectious that is causes huge epidemics and it is spread by water contamination.

It can be said that we had an advantage because of distance. Australia as an island situated a long way from the rest of the world.

*Parasitic Worms (Threadworms)* the more common worms such as the threadworms were seen in many of the children admitted, (*not the reason for admission-all simply part of admission procedure*) and were simply a matter of identification and standard medicinal treatment (Piperazine) with attention to hand cleanliness.

(*Roundworms*) were occasionally seen and certainly more serious, however not necessarily a reason for admission. The symptoms can resemble appendicitis, intestinal infection and even pneumonia. This is more a disease diagnosed in a general practice.

(*Tapeworms)* is a parasitic disease that was not usually admitted to Fairfield as a primary cause. Not because of lack of severity but mainly because the patient would be more inclined to be visiting a general practitioner over a period of time for vague symptoms and progressively becoming worse. Usually referred to a specialist and often resulting in an admission to a General Hospital Medical Ward.

The tapeworm lives in the intestines of animals including humans. Dogs are a popular host. They are also found in sheep country, therefore the need to cook meat extremely well particularly sheep and pork.

Hydatids disease resulting from the infestation is particularly serious as it grows in major organs, liver and lungs being a home to the Tapeworm-Hydatids.

Treatment requires getting the head otherwise the worm will grow again.

During the 1950's to 1965's we did not have the stringent requirements in the agricultural sector we do today. Milk and meat could cause serious illnesses if the agricultural preventative treatments were not strictly adhered to at all times.

(*Hookworm)* to the best of my knowledge we did not have a problem in this country or at least I do not remember a case of hookworm. I have been in lectures where students were made aware of the method of contracting hookworm.

My recollection was that when travelling overseas particularly the Northern Asian areas, it was emphasised NOT to go barefooted or to take shoes off and stand in the soil as the eggs are in the soil and will burrow into one's foot.

In later years when I travelled I was very aware of not removing foot wear when visiting sacred sites even though one was encouraged to do so!

*CHAPTER 12*

## Pathology:

Fairfield Infectious Diseases Hospital had one of the finest equipped pathology departments at that time. During the late 1950's pathology became "The Sir McFarlane Burnett" research laboratory.

The experienced medical and laboratory staff became well known overseas as authorities who were extremely well versed in "Infectious Diseases-Exotic Diseases".

The hospital was well known both nationally and internationally as an institute that lead the way in research, diagnosing and treating patients who presented with serious illnesses.

Fairfield Hospital was also instrumental in the eventual eradication of so many childhood and adult illnesses.

The hospital played a major part in setting the scene for a National Prevention Program and creating awareness in Community Health.

### Radiology:

At Fairfield it was necessary to be self-sufficient as we were unable to transfer patients externally for treatments. All radiology needed to be undertaken on the grounds-within Fairfield Hospital therefor a modern Radiology Department was essential.

Chest X-Rays alone would have kept the department busy.

The patients with Tuberculosis required progress images and patients with a secondary condition, for instance pneumonia certainly kept radiology busy.

CHAPTER 13

### Administration:

There was a separate building that housed administration. The Medical Superintendent, the Director of Nursing (Matron) and other Specialist Administrators.

Nursing staff visited only when necessary, patients rarely.

The Administration Department was a hub of total management, Board Rooms, Accounting Departments, Record keeping sections and so on....a domain that fulfilled Council, State Government and Federal Government requirements and obligations.

The specific nature of the Institute required a certain degree of isolation and autonomy however it was a small community that could impact on the safety of Australians.

Medically it was a vital part of Australia's Health System. As an island and quite a distance to any of our global neighbours, we were in a situation where we could protect our borders.

Being totally surrounded by ocean allowed us the benefit of quarantine stations that were strategically placed around our major coastal ports and incoming airports.

Interestingly enough and in hindsight, I would like to comment on life without computers, mobile phones, scanners and "other" electronic technological gadgetry we have in today's world.

Amazingly, the management of our small city within a city enabled a proficient, effective method of communication that enabled progress both within Australia and many other parts of the world! We were world recognised.

### Lecture Rooms:

Fairfield Hospital was a training hospital, a vital part of The Royal Melbourne Hospital and Associated School of Nursing therefore adequate facilities were required to be used in the education program.

Classes were scheduled daily; a timetable was provided appropriate to the level of skill or training of the trainee nurses.

Medical students did a stint at Fairfield; Registered Nurses undertaking post graduate studies also attended lectures. We had visiting Red Cross and there were Nurse's Aides who also used the lecture rooms so it was a busy educational facility.

**Nurses Home**:

As a student (18-21 years) it was compulsory to live-in. A nurse was to be unmarried, female, not engaged. During the 1950's it was unheard of to have "partners". All one's attention was expected to be total dedicated to one's career The Nurses Home was situated at the back of the hospital. Behind and below us the grounds sloped down to the Yarra River.

The accommodation had Nurses (trainees), Staff Nurses and Sisters living in the Home. There was a code that we all needed to abide by.... the normal, thoughtful, courteous, quiet behaviour was expected but most important of all the time for "Lights Out" this was not negotiable!

*The "Night Staff Sisters" while conducting rounds of the wards from 10.00pm to 6.00am also conducted rounds of the Nursing Home!*

*Unimaginable now in 2015!*

If nursing staff were on days off we were to be back by 10pm, sign in at the front gate and make our way by footpath to the Nurses Home quietly and speedily.

It may seem archaic now but it was an incredible way to keep control of a large number of 18 to 21 year aged females.

There were older ladies, "Nursing Sisters" of course but they were excluded from the young one's rules.

The rules and regulations worked, the authority that was wielded was often challenged by trainees. Even though the strength shown was noted the power held was tangible.

*It certainly did not leave any lasting fear of authority or cause any damage to one's confidence, but the firmness and control definitely instilled respect for authority.*

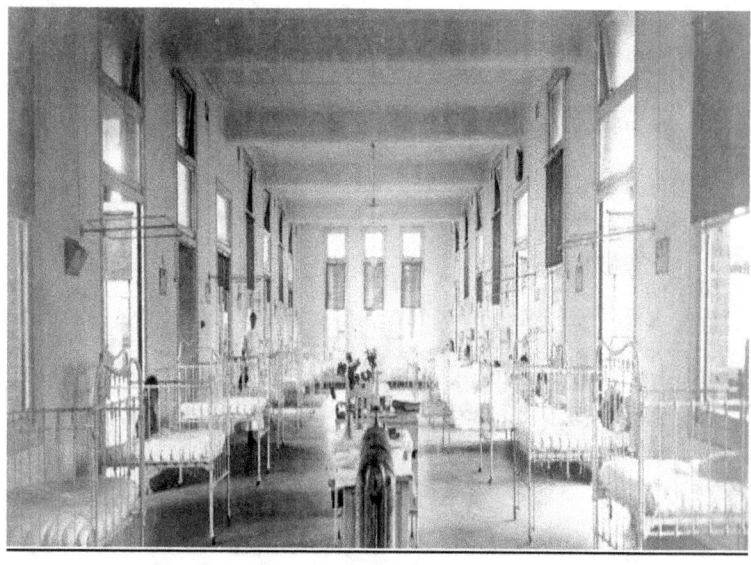

**A typical bright, light, airy ward at Fairfield Hospital**
(Photo courtesy Darebin Libraries Victoria)

CHAPTER 14

**CROSS-INFECTION:**

The subject of infection and cross-infection is an enormously important one. The seriousness of a person being admitted to hospital is in itself a stressful time for both patient and family but the thought of a secondary infection is totally unacceptable.

The amazing part of our training at Fairfield Hospital was the successful method of communicating *"What is Cross-Infection"* and *"How does it happen"?*

The lecturers were able to prepare a teaching program that spelt out the seriousness of cross-infection. The program was presented in a way that theoretically made sense and there was a component of the lectures that emphasized visually a "picture of how it happens".

At the time we were there as students we all agreed that the word "INFECTION" became a picture painted in our mind and there for ever. To this day I often foresee situations where infection is likely to occur and usually does.

The lecturers including pathologists were able to convey the message they were endeavouring to get across. They managed to imprint visual images.

Media was not very sophisticated in the 1950's so the method used to convey visual images was a little between pencil drawings, colourful paint, cartoons and comedic situations used to illustrate THE RIGHT WAY and THE WRONG WAY of approaching the nursing of infectious patients. The comic relief went down a treat!

Infection can be spread in so many ways most peculiar to the specific disease.

Air-borne disease can be spread by coughing, nasal discharge, sputum and sneezing.

Contact spread can be through pustules, sweat, nasal discharge, vomitus, and other bodily discharge.

Contamination can also be through, blood, urine, faeces and sloughing from wounds.

***Personal hygiene*** regarding the nurses was closely monitored. We were to wear our hair back of our face, finger nails were to be kept short, and nail polish was prohibited. Jewellery was not allowed including ear rings, hand rings and necklaces. Watches were to be pinned on our left chest.

These rules were carefully monitored.

Regardless of the method of transfer there is a basic standard of hygiene that all who make contact with patients must abide. Hand washing both before and after coming in contact with a patient is essential.

We, as students were not to wear our uniforms off the hospital grounds and we were to remove our aprons before going to the dining room. In the hospital wards, gowns were worn over our uniforms in many instances; however in the Block we gowned up on entry to each individual room.

*Objects* such as toys were not to be passed from child to child in fact most toys were not to leave Fairfield although some were suitable for sterilizing. Clothes worn by patients were all hospital clothes for the ease of laundering.

Reading material was not to be removed, on discharge of the patient and to minimize cross-infection, books were not to be transferred to different wards.

Food, utensils and scraps were emptied and food disposed of in the kitchens attached to each ward. Crockery and cutlery were washed then steam sterilized in the kitchens. Food was brought to each ward in "Hot Boxes" and served from the passage way onto trays which were taken to the patient.

*Laundry* was changed daily and placed in canvas bags, left at the exits for collection, they were then transferred to the on-site laundries.

Clean laundry was delivered on trolleys to the wards at the beginning of each morning.

After patients were discharged or transferred, the mattresses were placed out on the verandas where they were positioned to get maximum benefit of sterilization from the sun's rays. The beds were completely scrubbed with a strong disinfectant like Phenyl or Lysol and left outside on the veranda for 24 hours. Pillows went to the laundry.

*Furniture* was wiped over with disinfectant and stainless steel was wiped over with methylated spirits.

All doors, window sills, visitors' chairs and reachable walls were wiped regularly. Floors were washed daily with disinfectant, sweeping was **not allowed** as the theory was "the dust is simply flicked from one place to another", only wiping with moist-wet mops was allowed.

*Utensils-Equipment* was all cleaned in the sterilising rooms attached to each ward. There were large 4 x 3 x 6 feet deep (approximately) stainless steel containers in each ward with boiling water kept on simmer.

We washed instruments and treatment trays in soap and water in the troughs then immersed them into the sterilisers for a set time to sterilise.

The routine was an incredibly well thought out preventative method of minimising cross-infection......and IT WORKED.

The procedures were not time wasting. They were efficient, effective, tried and proven methods of establishing routines and procedures for ALL to follow.

I cannot speak highly enough of the "Powers that Be" at that time. Nothing was left to chance; every move was planned and scripted, to set a pattern for those that followed to strictly adhere to without question.

*"During my time at Fairfield Hospital as a Nurse in-training and my time, at a later date, as a Nursing Sister undertaking post-graduate studies, I at no time heard of a cross-infection or an instance where it could be said that a patient arrived with one disease and contracted another whilst in hospital".*

*Unfortunately in the last three decades this is not a statement that could be made by any hospital in Australia, to the best of my knowledge.*

*Coughing, sneezing and dirty hands all leave germs behind.*

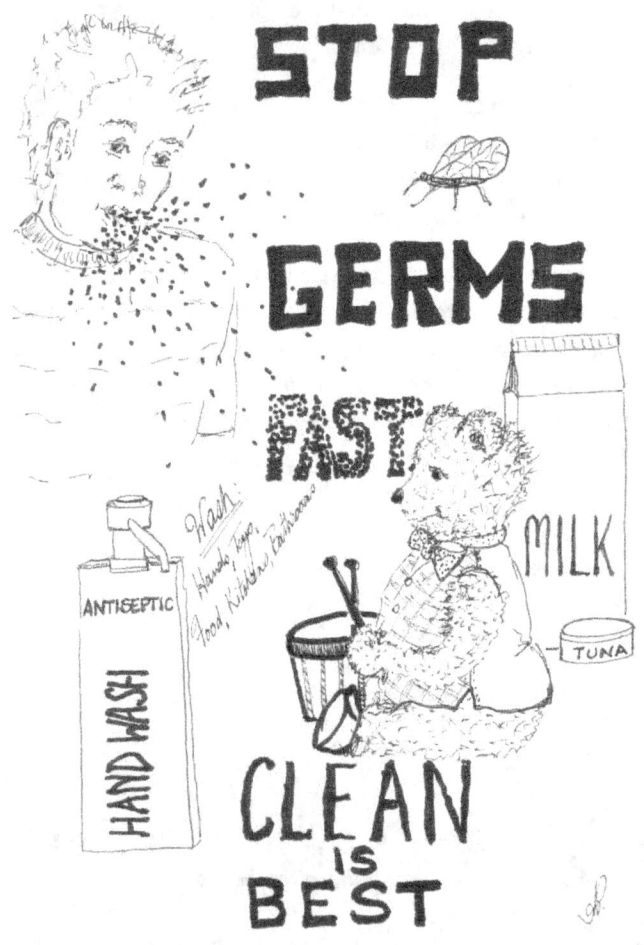

CHAPTER 15

### Outlining - Barrier Nursing

It is my belief that not only is "Barrier Nursing" rarely heard of outside of a hospital much less spoken about or indeed understood.

It is also my belief that the current dress code is less than compatible with what is required to prevent cross-infection.

**Now days it is my observation that the wearing of jewellery, the increase in long painted nails and indifference awarded to hair management is lax to the extent of non-existent.**

For the reduction of the spread of infection strict protocols must be put into place. Every person in the team must understand the basics to appreciate the overall reasons.

Infectious conditions are many and varied, therefore the general rule must be to assume you could contact the "germ" a number of ways. So prohibitively one covers "Street clothes" with a gown, prevent inhalation by wearing a mask, washing hands before touching the patient to prevent infection by contact.

Unfortunately the seriousness is not addressed even though statistically the evidence demonstrates the increase in cross-infection is at times out of control.......**WHY, I would ask?**

"Barrier nursing" also refers to a method we used when giving care to patients suffering from highly infectious diseases. This method was used to protect the other patients and everyone around from getting the disease. Those attending the patient wore masks and gowns as well as gloves for protection.

To prevent even a simple cold aspects of "Barrier Nursing" can be used simply to prevent cross-infection.

Modified, it is a method that can be used in the schools, work-place and even at home.

Most aspects are common sense:

- If coughing cover mouth
- If sneezing cover nose
- Do not share a handkerchief
- If tissues, dispose of without fingering
- Do not share food or drink vessels
- Do not sit on a patient's bed
- When talking keep a distance ....minimum one metre
- Keep travelling in public to a minimum
- Wash hands before eating
- Keep hands away from face, mouth, nose

The above list highlights a few precautions. Much can be done by thinking carefully and showing consideration to oneself as well as others.

*CHAPTER 16-SUMMARY*

Australia as an island is protected by sea however in the 1950-60's it was also protected from the rest of the world by distance. Therefore it took time for overseas people to get to our shores. During that time, many diseases were incubating during the long journey and patients were just beginning to show symptoms on arrival, therefore illness was usually reported not long after arrival. We managed to be prepared for diseases not previously experienced. It became obvious quickly on the patients arrival and we were prepared.

Over the last few decades the world has become a smaller place and with the speed of modern transport it is possible to bring unwanted diseases into Australia. The patient incubating disease is often out and about in the community spreading the disease as they move around!

From the 1950's on, in my experience we waited "with baited breath" for immunization, it came. We accessed whatever was on offer appreciatively knowing the misery of before!

Eventually in Australia we as near to...eradicated all major infectious diseases through immunisation.

I have shared my thoughts of Fairfield Hospital both as a young nurse training to a graduate nurse undertaking further studies.

Fairfield is the place I chose to undertake further studies prior to commencing one year full-time Midwifery studies.

I loved the atmosphere, the entire learning environment and the difference to elsewhere because of the specific nature of infectious diseases.

I remember with amazement the wonderful job Australia and Australians did by working together to enable eradication of many serious infectious diseases.

*What an incredible feat, particularly considering all the sceptics who needed to be convinced to come on board!*

I remember the Sanatoriums being turned into Rehabilitation facilities as we no longer had need to fill Sanatoriums with patient's with tuberculosis (TB) .

*Our last Polio cases were during the 1970's when mumps measles, diphtheria, small pox, tetanus, tuberculosis and chicken-pox were eradicated and other diseases either eradicated or reduced to a manageable level.*

*Amazing.......*

My experiences clearly demonstrate the measures taken in the 1950's to eliminate killer diseases. Today it would come under the heading of "Tough love" a method which has many critics.

The methods taken in the 1950-60's beginning with, public education together with compulsory Chest X-rays almost eliminated Tuberculosis. There would have been over 96% success rate.

*Compulsory Immunisation* programs for babies, pre-schooler children and primary school aged children, prevented outbreaks of so many communicable diseases.

Eventually came the closure of Fairfield Infectious Diseases Hospital in the 1990's. The facility was modified for a totally different Government requirement and is currently used for that need in 2014.

During the period I have referred to in the book, the public didn't question authority as much as they have done in more recent times.

Whether it is right or wrong to be more conscious of one's rights, is not for me to say, however in the field of communicable diseases it certainly is not in the interest of the general public to question **FACTS**.....that is quiet obvious!

**Scientists worked with such commitment and passion to discover drugs that would give us protection from disabling or killer diseases. Finally immunisation became available for prevention of many diseases and it has proved its effectiveness over a period of at least fifty years that I can recall....**

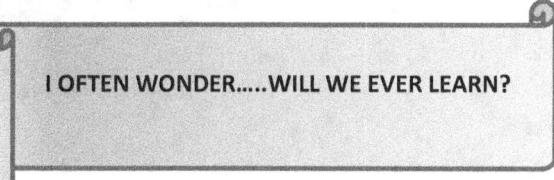

I OFTEN WONDER.....WILL WE EVER LEARN?

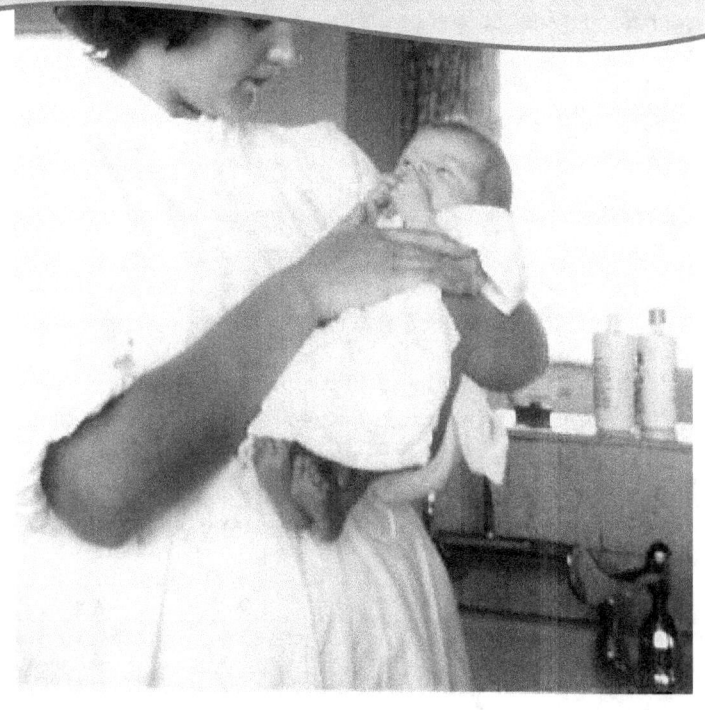

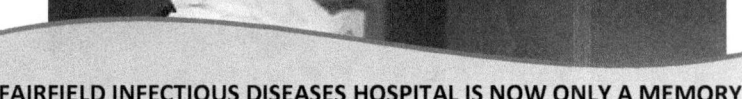

FAIRFIELD INFECTIOUS DISEASES HOSPITAL IS NOW ONLY A MEMORY OF A PREVIOUS ERA